PRAISE FOR

Stop Thinking About It!

"Stop Thinking About It! has an extremely important message that I agree with wholeheartedly, and it has made a positive difference in my life."   – Fay K.

"These concepts are liberating. I no longer feel trapped."
                                                                          – Sarah H.

"Stop Thinking About It! is a quick read that yields big results."
                                                                          – Terina E.

"Your story resonated so well with me, I kept thinking, 'That's me!' I can't wait to start applying the steps."
                                                                          – Caralee A.

"Thank you for writing *Stop Thinking About It!* It has changed the issue from saying 'No' to foods our culture tells me I want, to saying 'Yes' to what my body *truly* wants. I have finally made real change."   – Carol F.

Stop Thinking About It!

Stop Thinking About It!

Winning the Emotional Battle
Surrounding Food and Weight Loss

LORI A. WILLIAMS

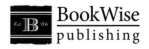

Stop Thinking About It:
Winning the Emotional Battle Surrounding Food and Weight Loss

BookWise Publishing
Salt Lake City, Utah
www.bookwisepublishing.com

www.stopthinkingaboutit.com

Book design by Eden Graphics, Inc., Salt Lake City, Utah
Illustrations by Elliott

Stop Thinking About It:
Winning the Emotional Battle Surrounding Food and Weight Loss
Williams, Lori A.

ISBN: 978-1-60645-073-4
Library of Congress Control Number: 2011902408
10 9 8 7 6 5 4 3 2 1
First Printing

Printed in the USA

For those women and men, girls and boys,

who have tried to diet, tried to be healthy,

tried to lose weight—

and have been left feeling unsuccessful,

frustrated, and consumed by the effects of food.

May you find great hope in my message.

Table of Contents

Introduction

I realize that I am putting myself in a rather vulnerable position in telling the following experiences, but I'm compelled to share.

I am a thirty-five year old woman, married to a wonderful man, and we have been blessed with six delightful children. I feel healthy; I am happy, and my mind is free from the emotional burden that food, diets, and a critical self-image often bring. However, I've not always been so fortunate. The freedom I now feel is a gift that came after years of feeling just that—burdened. I firmly believe that this gift is available to all who consider what I have to say. My message is simple: **Stop thinking about it!**

I remember exactly when I became so aware of *me*. In junior high, I made specific note of another girl's legs. Now hear me out. Her legs were simply thin and strong, and I accepted the notion that I would be happier if only my legs were like hers too. I wasn't overweight, but for the first time I became critically aware of what I *believed* I needed to look like in order to be happy.

Of course, if I wanted to change the way I was going to look, I was going to have to change the way I ate and exercised. So I made a plan. When could I eat or not eat? When could I have treats? How was I going to get stronger? What would I have to change? Thus began my burden.

I decided right away that I was going to have to cut out treats, and I needed to exercise regularly. I began to pay better attention to the foods I ate and learned more about healthy options. I thought a lot about it. For the next few years, I had plan after plan—diet after diet— that I hoped would bring me the results I wanted. Some brought better results than others did. With each new effort I began with the idea that I would start my new, healthy habits *tomorrow*. Tomorrow would come with the determination that I was not going to eat any treats. Nope, no treats, just for a day or maybe even a week. I could do it.

After one particular school day, I told myself that I was only going to have a sandwich as a snack. I knew that a big bag of cookies was in the refrigerator, but I thought about it and reminded myself that I was not going to have any. I would have self-control. *Yep. I can do it. No problem. No cookies*, I told myself. But from there I proceeded to think about the cookies every few minutes. The more I thought about them, the more I wanted one. In no time, I found myself eating a cookie, and then another, and another . . . Whatever happened to my resolve and self-control? Of course, after

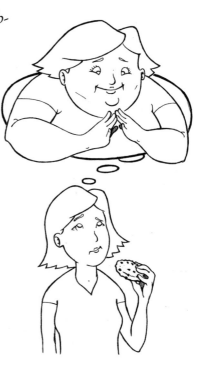

eating several, I chastised myself, rehearsing that I knew better. I was going to get wider for sure. In fact, I was gaining weight as I sat there! And after so many cookies, I didn't feel well either. *Exercise!* I thought to myself. *I could go and do some exercise.* That's right. My guilt was such that I decided to work out *on a full stomach.*

I have seven sisters and three brothers. My father was very protective of his girls. One of his rules was that we were not to go jogging alone outside of our cul-de-sac. Even a group of two was not generally enough; three was preferred. So here I was concerned about all the cookies I ate and was ready to exercise *right away.*

My options were slim. After thinking it over, running seemed like my best bet, but my father's rules were quite restrictive. I was intent, however, on feeling better (emotionally and physically) about those cookies. So off I went, around the cul-de-sac, again and again, guessing how many laps would equal a mile, and getting dizzy on a full stomach. Nice. Sadly, this *type* of occurrence was not an isolated adolescent incident.

It was during those years that I became interested in

nutrition. My willpower was actually quite strong during certain phases. During one such phase, I restricted myself to three treats a week. I allowed one on Monday, one on Wednesday, and one on the weekend. I stuck with this successfully for quite a while, but I could not keep it up forever. Diets worked for a short time, after which I would quickly gain back the pounds I'd lost with such great effort.

After a few years, I found myself over-thinking meals. At one point I would eat, then immediately begin thinking about my next snack or meal. I was keenly aware of how long it had been since I last ate, and when it would be okay to eat again. Disappointment lingered as I had waited all that time, and the meal was over so quickly. At other times, I woke in the morning with my first thoughts centered on breakfast. I did not eat to live—I lived to eat.

This mindset was consuming. I constantly created new dietary plans, failed to live up to my expectations, and felt guilty. It was a vicious cycle that

I did not eat to live. I lived to eat.

resulted in a persistent cloud of discontent.

This moderate, yet nagging emotional battle went on for several years. I figured the only way to be completely satisfied was to push through some form of food regulation again with the hope of next time having greater willpower and more energy of mind. This was exhausting and ultimately discouraging.

Don't misunderstand. I don't mean to paint a doom and gloom picture of my mentality. I was like most girls, busy with school, friends, work, and family. I enjoyed learning, having new experiences, and being social. I was generally happy. I would definitely highlight my teenage years as a great time in my life. However, I think that most women (and many men) can identify to one degree or another with this constant fog that reminds us of food and its effects. It was tough to shake.

In reviewing a recent study conducted by psychology professor, Diane Spangler, and graduate student, Tyler Owens, Sara Israelsen-Hartley found that, "the brains of healthy, well-adjusted women with no history of eating disorders were activated in a similar way to bulimics when shown pictures of overweight women."

Mark Allen, a Brigham Young University neuro-scientist, says, "At a subconscious level, they really are bothered by the prospect of [gaining weight]."[1] Many men are not exempt either. This subconscious aware-ness of how we look seems to linger in the back of our minds, and it affects us even when we don't realize it.

After many years of feeling burdened by discon-tentment, I've come across an emotionally and physi-cally healthy approach to achieving the peace of mind I craved. I've lived it for several years, and it works. I've shared these thoughts about my early experiences in hopes that those who identify with the same burden might, too, have hope and, ultimately, peace of mind. My solution is straightforward, natural, costs nothing, and just makes sense—*stop thinking about it*.

CHAPTER 1

Stop Thinking About It!

I've always been taught self-control, but what about those moments when your self-control fails you, as it applies to the "dos" and "don'ts" of healthy eating? It seems that every diet I've come across has thoroughly expressed what not to eat, then asks that you measure your food, analyze your food, and deny yourself food. Food, food, food. Diets are primarily about pipe dreams of massive weight loss if you just . . . They ramp up your emotions with hopes of a celebrity body if you just . . . They capture your heart with the idea that their plan is actually a revolutionary weight loss breakthrough fix if you just . . . In the long term, do these diets really work? *No.* Who has that kind of self-discipline—really? Diets expect you to be conscious of foods, and yet not eat them. It's like tantalizing you with what you really want and then saying, "But you can't have it." You're expected to eat irregularly for the rest of your life, which suggests never-ending emotional battles.

Many of us can be successful on a diet for a short period of time, but when we stop, we are so aware of what we've been suppressing, that all we want is a lot of what we haven't had. We usually end up overeating and gaining

> It's like tantalizing you with what you really want and then saying, "But you can't have it."

back what we've lost, and then some. Our heightened awareness of what we are restricting—food—ends up beating us in the end.

So, **STOP THINKING ABOUT IT!**

Stop dieting, stop worrying, and start living. *Don't be surprised when you LOSE WEIGHT too.*

As you go through your day and find yourself thinking about how you would really like some cookies, don't reason through why you should deny yourself them.

Don't tell yourself that you will regret eating them. Don't stew about the forty pounds you're planning on losing. Redirect your thoughts to something else instead. Later, when you think a soda would be great instead of water, occupy your thoughts with other interests. At lunch, when you have a couple of cookies for dessert and you kick yourself for being so weak, don't beat yourself up. Drop the thought and move on.

Don't think about food unless you are planning dinner, buying groceries, preparing a meal, or eating. When you have finished eating, don't think about your next meal. If you ate too much, don't beat yourself up.

Thoughts are powerful. They are the control center for your action and attitude, thereby playing a significant role in what you do and feel.

All Action is born in Thought

You can only think one thought at

a time, so force another thought into food's place. Have a replacement ready if you struggle with this at first. Think of a song. Rehearse something funny you heard recently. Count the paper clips in your desk. *Anything* else will help. If you're able, *do* something different entirely. Don't give up. You will gradually think about food less and less. It will become easier and easier to drop unwanted thoughts.

Every action is preceded by a thought. You don't just do things without having considered them first. Choosing what you eat is no exception. Before anything makes its way into your stomach, you first think about it. Then you judge whether you're going to eat it. Finally, you either put it in your mouth or turn it down. The removal of the first step cuts out even the possibility of eating it. In other words, when you think about food less, you eat less. As such, a maintained weight or weight loss will become a natural side effect. *Can it be that simple? Can weight management really start with your fleeting thoughts? Absolutely!*

> **Everything we do begins with a thought.**

Please understand there is a big difference between *not thinking about food* and *guilt-free eating*. Will you miraculously get thin if you throw caution to the wind and eat anything you'd like? No. You'll gain, not lose. You need to take your mind off food *before* you casually overeat, not just afterward. Can you enjoy your favorite unhealthy food guilt-free occasionally? Yes. Should you make a batch of brownies whenever you feel the urge? No. When the desire comes to buy (or bake) your favorite treat (or junk food) after you've just done the same the day before, remind yourself to stop thinking about what is tempting you. Simply think about something else. Better yet, go do something unrelated to help take your mind off food.

> When you think about food less, you eat less.

It is up to you to gauge how often you should enjoy your "forbidden" comfort foods. I tend to think that one should be able to go a couple of days, comfortably, without those dishes that currently seem to tempt. To some, that may sound easy, but for most I suspect going a day without dessert of one kind or another is tough. It was certainly difficult for me. Now, sometimes I'll comfortably go several days without a treat. I pass up desserts often because they truly don't sound good to me. Occasionally, a dessert will really just hit the spot, but more often than not, treats don't even taste exciting.

Over time, I began to crave "useful" foods that made me feel good because they fueled me. In my experience, food is only abused when it is used for something other than fuel. So for starters, STOP thinking about it.

I remember a time when I was in high school and was trying hard—thinking so hard—to eat healthy foods. My family was roasting s'mores in the backyard fire pit. I loved the tasty combination of warm marshmallows, melted chocolate, and graham crackers. With my determination to eat healthy, I knew that I shouldn't have one, but I struggled to pass it up. I formulated a plan. If I made something similar that wasn't as bad for me, I wouldn't feel guilty. So I proceeded to mix a roasted marshmallow with raw oats and stirred. It didn't stir. It clumped and stuck, but I ate it anyway. Gross. It was neither good nor satisfying. I sat in the house with my bowl of marshmallow oats that night, thinking about everyone outside by the fire enjoying themselves.

I wasted my evening worrying about the love/hate relationship I had with food. I stewed over it for a while and eventually gave in to eating a real s'more. In the end, I could do nothing productive until I satisfied my craving. Then I proceeded to feel disappointed in my lack of willpower.

On another occasion I chose to pass on a favorite dessert. My desire for that chocolate cake rolled around in my head for an hour after dinner, and I struggled to get past it. I found myself going back to the kitchen in search of something else to satisfy my craving. To avoid the cake, I ate a hunk of leftover white rice. (You know how rice takes the shape of the bowl after it cools? Yes, a hunk of rice.) I wasn't happy that night. I was frustrated and unsatisfied. This type of emotional battle was common for me then. Routinely, it consumed my thinking.

Let's fast forward through high school to college and past several years of marriage, as well as multiple pregnancies. After many years of having a heightened awareness of food and its effects, I made a conscious decision to keep either from my mind unless necessary. Surprisingly enough, in the absence of those useless thoughts, my interest in food changed and, with that, my actions did too. I began to eat when I was *hungry*, not just because I wanted to. I recognized that thoughts were the precursor to my actions.

Making this simple adjustment was the first step in making proper decisions concerning what my body needed for nourishment instead of battling self-control and dieting at every turn. With this I shifted my energy from how I looked to how I felt. I identified new "quick joy." I continued to try to eat plenty of healthy foods and being active remained a priority.

> Following this process allowed my mind to make proper decisions concerning what my body needed for nourishment instead of battling self-control and dieting at every turn.

This was a gradual process; it wasn't overnight. In fact, over a period of weeks or months (I'm not exactly sure), it occurred to me that I wasn't uptight about what I ate anymore, and my critical awareness of my "shape" was drastically lower. My mind was free from these burdens and available for other things. It may be worth mentioning that I'm now the lightest I've been in years. Weight loss came naturally as a result of the changes I'm recommending. My experience was not completely revolutionary. This was simply a series of principles that, when working together, created an amazing result. Each section of this book was a step in my journey.

As an interesting side note, I have felt the constant pull from food as I've spent time compiling my thoughts on this matter. Food has been on my mind much more now that I've been rehashing the process I went through to be emotionally free of it. I've left each writing session with a craving for junk food. In fact, as I'm writing this, I'm eating a piece of cake that isn't even good. It was just available. It's been sitting in the freezer for three weeks, never tempting me until now while I'm thinking about food.

The other day, as I closed the notebook in which I was compiling my thoughts, I wanted ice cream. Following another writing session, I felt desperately hungry. My mind began to slip back into its old ways. I felt again, briefly, the emotional burden I used to know so well. Ouch! Walk away from the worry! I had to remind myself to STOP thinking about it. Ah. Peace again. The mind is a powerful tool.

It's been said many times when dedicating oneself to a nutritional plan of action, "I just need to make it a way of life." What you're really saying is, "I can do it. I just have to deprive myself of something I will want terribly for the rest of my life." I have yet to meet anyone with this kind of willpower. I certainly don't have it.

> It is allowing "moderation in all things" to occur without the fight.

What I am suggesting is an approach that is healthy for your body *and* mind. It is allowing "moderation in all things" to occur without the fight. I've done this for several years. Because it cuts to the core of the issue, it's sustainable. It's balanced. It works.

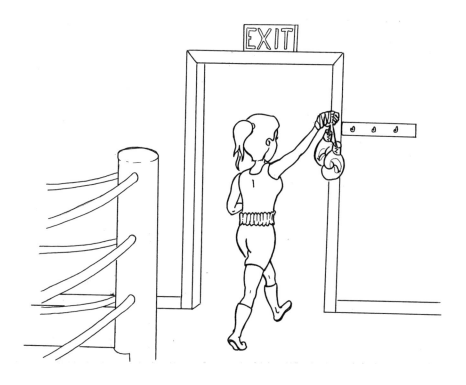

Summary: Stop thinking about food. Drop your thoughts about food unless you are planning dinner, buying groceries, preparing a meal, or eating. The goal is to take the emotional battle out of healthy eating.

CHAPTER 2

How Do You Feel?

Do you spend more energy thinking about how you look or how you feel? There is a big difference. Many of us get caught up in thinking that we can't be happy unless we have a celebrity body. Not true. We think that looking "hot" is the missing link to a life of joy, and anything less equals sadness. Everyone is searching for happiness. However, allowing such a large portion of our happiness to be determined by our body shape is a huge burden for anyone to carry. A passionate quest for this ideal shape often leads to frustration, discouragement, and weight gain. My suggestion is that we concern our-selves less with our weight and place more interest on how we feel. In other words, stop worrying about whether or not that piece of chocolate cake will make you put on the pounds. In-stead, pay better attention to the way your body feels after eating it.

> **Worry less about how you look, and more about how you physically feel.**

In Chapter One, we talked about cutting a lot of un-necessary eating by thinking about food less. However, we do have to eat sometime. We cannot avoid thinking about food completely. So for those thoughts of food that must stick around, we must next choose what to eat. If we are to avoid an emotional battle, it is necessary that we re-train our brain to think about food differently.

When we better discern how our body feels in response to food, two things occur. First, we shift our thoughts away from something that tends to control us (the emotional battle that surrounds food choices and a critical body image), replacing this with positive emo-tions we can feel every day (simply feeling energetic and fueled). Second, becoming more aware of how foods make us feel physically gives us invaluable experience that naturally promotes change in our eating habits, leading to a healthier, happier person. *This is big.*

When I refer to the emotional battle, I'm talking about the battle that many of us allow into our heads, playing good versus evil. Who will win today and then what? I allude to our interest in losing weight, trying to diet, succeeding or failing, worrying about it, overeating to cover painful emotions, trying harder, wanting it *more*, getting upset when we are weak, worrying about how we look, and so on. We want something badly, but that part of us inside that doesn't want to sacrifice for it is set in opposition against that part of us that is trying hard to have the willpower it requires. This recurrent conflict is emotionally draining.

The idea of shifting our thoughts away from the emotional battle and, instead, toward how our body feels in response to food is key. Sometimes it's a temptation to worry about our physical imperfections, but dropping those thoughts and enjoying the feeling of being energized after eating a healthy meal offers immediate satisfaction. We have the opportunity to feel that satisfaction every day, at every meal. So concern yourself less with how you look and more with how you physically feel.

The other day I told my aunt about how I don't suffer with the food-centered emotional battle anymore. She expressed to me that such a thing is a great blessing and agreed that this critical physical awareness is something that women of all ages worry about. She explained that because of her physical response to allergies, it was easier to avoid certain foods that weren't good for her simply because they made her sick. Again, it was because of her negative reaction to those foods that it became easier to avoid them. In this regard, her allergies actually lent a positive result. This is the same principle behind paying better attention to how foods make us feel. If the effect can be felt with certain allergies, why can't it work with everything we eat?

Most people pay little attention to their specific physical response to foods they eat, but rather are wrapped up in how it makes them feel emotionally. Teach yourself to care more about how your body feels physically by paying better attention to its messages.

How do you feel physically as you go through your day? Take note. You may be surprised at how great a role food choice plays. How do you feel when you eat a donut for breakfast? You may experience a great emotional sensation for a minute, but before long what is your physical response? Not good. *Note to self: my body feels heavy and tired.* Don't beat yourself up, just move on.

> Teach yourself to care more about how your body feels physically by paying better attention to its messages.

You go out to lunch at an all-you-can-eat buffet and have some very tasty food. Yes, it's delicious. You keep going back for more because you just can't pass it up. But how does your body feel a little later?

At dinner, you're quite hungry so you fill your plate. Even though your body triggered that it was full before you had finished your food, you cleaned your plate because you hate to waste. What is your physical response?

Note to self: I feel too full. In fact, I'm uncomfortable, and it's hard to focus on other things. We've all probably felt that again and again. The same could be said for an afternoon snack from the vending machine. *Note to self: a delayed reaction to the candy was feeling drained.*

Your body wants to be fueled with healthy foods— healthy being for the overall good health and longevity of your body. Paying better attention to how your body responds to what you eat puts the influence of your food choices on what your *body* wants, not on what your *mind* wants. Incidentally, your body doesn't want junk food; this is all your mind's doing.

You may begin leaving the last two or three bites on your dinner plate. Perhaps you'll subconsciously ask yourself, "Why would I eat the last couple of bites at the cost of feeling uncomfortable?" Skipping the donuts in the office break room will be easier because you just don't want to feel that "post-donut feeling." You may find yourself craving eggs or whole grain cereal for breakfast instead of Fruit Loops. Don't be surprised if you begin to turn down desserts because you actually don't want them. You might be hungry for a snack and actually prefer a handful of almonds to candy or a bag of chips.

Once I adapted to paying better attention to my body's physical cues, healthier food had never looked so good.

> Once I adapted to paying better attention to my body's physical cues, healthier food had never looked so good.

I have compiled a series of my mental "notes to self." My hope is that sharing some of these might be helpful. As you practice listening to your body, what you notice may not be exactly like me. What you learn about yourself is specific to *you*.

MY "NOTES TO SELF"

Foods high in preservatives leave me feeling shaky, almost sick. I can feel the difference, for example, when I eat a pre-made rice dish and one from scratch. The other day I was eating ice cream. It was one of my favorite brands. It was natural, free of preservatives, and I felt content when I'd finished. On a different occasion, I was offered an ice cream sandwich that was filled with a variety of unnatural ingredients. I accepted. Halfway into it, I felt weak and tired and chose not to finish it. Our bodies function better after eating natural foods. As we become more in tune with how our body feels in response to how we feed it, food choices become easier because unhealthy options actually become less desirable.

Fast food leaves me feeling de-energized and . . . just bad. Occasionally, I think it would be nice to enjoy a quick burger like I did years ago, but

I don't want to feel that way—that ugh—that yucky feeling that I can't quite find words for. If you don't know what I am talking about, next time you enter that drive-through, pay closer attention. What's your body's reaction to a burger and fries? Once in a long while, I'll order it, too, and I quickly remember why I stopped. It's not worth having that feeling.

Deep fried foods seem to penetrate every part of me. I feel greasy all over, inside and out. It seems as if the grease floats right up to the surface of my skin. Come to think about it, my skin does reflect what I eat, so maybe there's some truth to this.

I get tired soon after I consume a lot of sugar. When I eat candy, for example, my blood glucose level raises quickly, forcing insulin to be released from my pancreas. This insulin quickly lowers my blood sugar, and I feel tired. Candy corns—need I say more?

Drinking water doesn't disturb my vitality or appetite like others drinks do. When eating a meal, I prefer water. Other drinks that have sugar or carbonation mess with the flavor and digestion of my meal.

Green salads with varied veggies, beans, nuts, whole grains, and dressing leave me feeling happier, energized and fueled. I think I'm literally a happier person after I eat a great, multi-ingredient salad. My eyes open a little wider, my zeal for life surfaces, and my productivity is greater. It's almost as if my body is saying, "Thank you!"

Fruit is sweet and refreshing. Years ago I set a goal that I was not going to eat any treats for a whole month. That would be a first for me and the task was daunting, but I was determined in my resolve to do as I'd set out. It was torture for a couple of weeks, and I didn't know how I was ever going to make it. Broken for a time from sugar, however, I developed a new appreciation for how sweet fresh fruit is. It tasted every bit as sweet as candy, and I could be content.

Eating whole grain bread leaves me feeling better than breads made with white flour. For college graduation I got a wheat grinder and couldn't have been happier. The ladies at work, on the other hand, didn't get it. A wheat grinder? For graduation? Yes. Great homemade bread was something I grew up with, and I had a patient mother who showed me the ropes. My appreciation for freshly ground wheat took root, and I knew a grinder would someday be a staple in my kitchen.

It's been many years since I got that grinder, and it's been put to good use. Yesterday, however, I made *white* bread dough, and with my children spun dough "snakes" around previously shaped tin foil molds to form tiny cornucopias for Thanksgiving. Out of the oven came all sorts of gnarled efforts. Despite their odd looks, we unraveled those babies one row at a time, and downed them. Of course, before long I felt the white-flour-feeling that's hard to describe. I got full, but didn't feel *fed*.

This morning I made waffles but didn't want to use white flour this time. They were made of 100% whole wheat and shaped like hearts. I know, shaped baking two days in a row for my children? I was so proud of myself I could hardly stand it. Anyhow, we ate them up as well, but there was a very distinct difference in how I felt later that morning, as compared to the previous day. I felt *fed*, not just sustained by calories. Whole grain. Your body knows the difference.

After I exercise I tend to crave more healthy foods. On those days when I go for a quick ten-minute run first thing in the morning, I don't care to follow it with a donut or sweet cereal. I want something more wholesome. Not only am I eating better in the morning, but what I eat for breakfast tends to set a standard for the rest of the day.

Exercising soon after eating is not fun and much harder than otherwise. My mind is drawn to those nights of running around the cul-de-sac after dinner due to overeating and regret. Ugh. Exercising first thing in the morning before I eat a full breakfast feels better.

It doesn't feel good to go to sleep on a full stomach. I feel much better when I avoid eating two or three hours before bedtime.

When I am between meals and need a snack, almonds take that hunger away and leave me feeling fueled. Since I've learned to respond to my body's physical cues, I actually find myself inconvenienced from time to time by the need to eat, so when I *do* eat, I'm more concerned with ridding hunger than counting calories.

A protein drink often satisfies my munchies.
Sometimes I find myself returning again and again to the pantry, craving something I can't put my finger on. Many snacks later, I still don't feel content. My body is confusing hunger for thirst or a vitamin/mineral deficiency. When I cut to the chase and fill my body's need, it is *then* that I am satisfied. I'll try a protein drink (protein), chickpeas (iron), cheese (calcium), or whatever I think I may need. A regular intake of vitamin supplements can help avoid these deficiencies (and thereby cravings) as well.

To further illustrate, allow me to share two examples that show our body's capacity to recognize our vitamin/mineral deficiencies. My brother-in-law suffers from Type 1 diabetes. A key role in dealing with this condition is managing his blood sugar levels. He has learned to recognize his body's reaction to high or low blood sugar and responds with foods that stabilize it. Similarly, pregnant women tend to have some very specific cravings as their body is depleting the mother's store of vitamins for creating a baby. Although these are extreme cases, they help demonstrate our body's ability to understand its dietary needs. We can *learn* to recognize these cues.

Eating junk food on an empty stomach makes me feel jittery. In comparison, when I have a solid meal or a healthy snack when I'm hungry, I feel fueled and energized. One good example of this principle occurred on a night when I had a meeting away from home. At its conclusion, I was very hungry and there were refreshments being served, including a variety of cookies and punch. I chose to turn them down, because I know how I feel after eating treats on an empty stomach. It wasn't worth that jittery feeling. I waited until I got home and had leftovers which made me satisfied and comfortable.

I can tell when I'm full within a few of bites of finishing a meal. My body will let me know when it no longer needs more. I often leave one or two bites on my plate because those next two bites are the difference between being fed and happy versus being overfed and unhappy. Similarly, there have been many times when I've let the last few bites of ice cream melt in my bowl to be tossed or saved for later. Those last few bites were the difference between enjoying the dessert and feeling uncomfortable. We all want to feel good, so why ruin it by overeating?

> Those last few bites were the difference between enjoying the dessert and feeling uncomfortable.

Some may dispute and say they simply don't have a built-in sensor. They can't feel the trigger that tells them they are full. If this strikes a chord with you, don't give up. Practicing the principles outlined in this book will increase your sensitivity to feeling full.

My experience suggests that knowing when to stop is a learned behavior.

When I'm not hungry and I eat, I don't feel good. It's like my body is saying, "Hold on. What's this for? I don't need to eat yet." This concept has been a huge help for me when it comes to declining the extra social food that the American culture promotes. Treats were hard for me to decline if they were out. Now, if I'm not really craving something, I can easily pass on them because they don't sound good to me.

We don't become overweight by eating. We become overweight by eating when we're not hungry or by eating too many unhealthy foods.

The other day I offered my two-year-old daughter a piece of cake. She declined. "No, don't want to." She had just eaten some lunch and wasn't interested. A little later, she asked for a banana. Now, my daughter certainly likes treats, but this time her body didn't want it, and she didn't have the emotional attraction swirling around in her head convincing her that she should eat it anyway simply because it was offered. What she really craved was a banana, something her body noted as fuel. Hmm. It would seem this mind game is a learned evil.

Remember that these are some of *my* examples. This is *my* body's response. Everyone is different, so you may experience different effects. Consider including other notes responding to your sleep needs, food combining, or anything else that comes to mind. How did *you* feel? Allow this to be an important question for you. Let *it* concern you more than your figure.

Don't forget that these reminders need to be administered guilt-free. They are notes, not lectures. Also, while being more aware of how foods make you physically feel is central to your success, this doesn't mean that you want it on your mind regularly. Recognize your reactions, but don't dwell on them. Your new under-standing will begin to influence your choices without much time or thought.

This is a gradual process. You don't become in tune with your body overnight. It takes time, but it's worth it. The emotional battle will gradually fade away through a natural redirection toward eating to live, not living to eat.

There's also another great side effect of this re-train-ing of your brain. When you follow your body's natural cues, you will not become overweight; and if you have weight to lose, you will begin to lose it.

Summary: Decide that you care more about how you feel than how you look. Teach yourself to become more aware of what food choices make you feel good and which ones make you feel not so good. You'll natu-rally care more about fueling your body instead of telling yourself what you should or shouldn't eat, thereby either losing weight, maintaining a healthy body or both.

———————— ⤬ ————————

CHAPTER 3

Understanding Your Balance

With the unlimited options we have available to us for food, you'd think it would be a cinch to nourish our bodies with well-rounded meals that satisfy and give us the energy we need. I'm guessing we've been told countless times to eat our fruits and vegetables and avoid sugar. I mean, how hard can it be? Just eat like we know we should. It's that simple, right?

Obviously, it's easier said than done. When judging what to eat, we subconsciously entertain thoughts from two influences—our *mind* and our *body*.

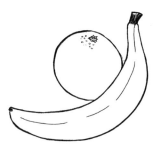

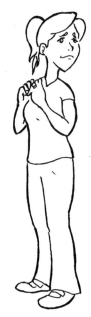

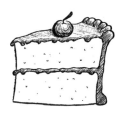

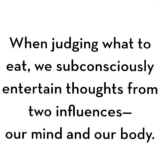

When judging what to eat, we subconsciously entertain thoughts from two influences— our mind and our body.

Our *mind* wants food that gives a positive emotional sensation. Often this "quick joy" is felt through foods that are high in sugar or salt. This category tends to be filled with unhealthy foods that are high in calories and low in lasting energy. The bottom line is that when the cookies are on the table, our desire to taste the pleasure offered has more pull than our concern over their lack of qualities that support good health.

Our *body*, on the other hand, craves that which benefits our health and stamina, leaving us feeling fueled.

Among these cravings, you'll notice lots of fruits, vegetables, whole grains, and the avoidance of junk food.

In Melinda Beck's *Wall Street Journal* article, "Eating to Live or Living to Eat?," she clarifies these two influences as hedonic (mind) and homeostatic (body). For hedonic eaters, "Seeing, smelling, and even hearing the word 'cake' activate areas of the brain involved in reward, emotion, memory and thinking, triggering the release of dopamine, the brain's 'pleasure chemical.'" For homeostatic eaters, "When food reaches the stomach and intestines, chemical messengers slow down digestion and signal to the brain to stop eating. Seeing cake isn't as tempting." [2]

The following example illustrates this principle. Upon returning to work from lunch, you feel energized and content. It is then you come across the box of donuts available in the break room. "Homeostatic" (body) eaters walk away empty-handed, while "hedonic" (mind) eaters ignore the regulator inside that communicates lack of hunger and struggle to pass up the perceived pleasure.

> "Hedonic" response: eating for pleasure. "Homeostatic" response: eating for survival.

The terms hedonic and homeostatic represent two different and distinct perspectives, but in reality everyone has a blend of both. The question is how much effect will these two influences have on your everyday eating? Each of us has a different balance.

Let's consider this balance in three individuals labeled person A, person B, and person C. To simplify, I'll continue with the terms *mind* and *body*.

Even though **Person A** knows that junk food is not healthy, the desire for a short-lived "joy" most often wins because they're programmed to pay greater heed to the emotional pleasure that comes from eating it. The *body's* willpower has a hard time arguing with what the *mind* desires. These two oppose each other, creating emotional battles on a regular basis. This person probably thinks about food a lot.

Person B might have a relatively healthy balance but may do so leaning heavily on their willpower. They are content and feel that they have the emotional battle under

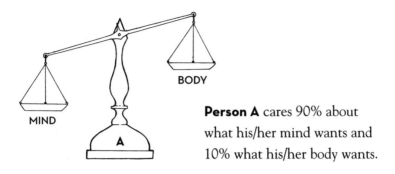

Person A cares 90% about what his/her mind wants and 10% what his/her body wants.

Person B cares 50% about what his/her mind wants and 50% what his/her body wants.

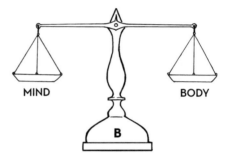

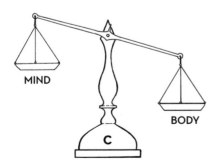

Person C cares 10% about what his/her mind wants and 90% what his/her body wants.

control, *control* being the operative word. While self-control is very important, most people would appreciate fewer circumstances that demand it.

The balance of **Person C** would suggest that they have few emotional battles surrounding food and weight loss. They tend to eat plenty of healthy foods because that's what they want, not because of increased will-power. This person enjoys unhealthy foods from time to time but they don't worry about it. They leave the last couple of bites of food on their plate if it means the difference between being comfortable and uncomfortable. This person successfully finds joy in varied quality of life pursuits because they are not burdened by the battle over food's version of good versus evil.

Though I've spent the last several years experiencing varied degrees of Person C's behaviors, I have undoubtedly felt all three of these levels of balance. The following illustrations demonstrate my mindset in each condition.

90% mind / 10% body:

As mentioned previously, at some point food became the common link to my day's activities. Upon waking in the morning, I was anxious to eat breakfast. Afterward, I was interested in planning lunch. Occasionally, I calculated how much time had to elapse before it would be okay to eat again. Any hint of a hunger pang would send me to the fridge. Disappointed that lunch was over so quickly, I looked forward to a snack or dinner.

During this time I tended to put a lot of hope in dieting, and the outcome seemed critical to my happiness. I ate healthy foods regularly, but with the amount of time I spent thinking about the joy of food, my efforts often failed because of the emotional battle required to succeed. With 90% of my choices driven by my emotional interests and only 10% led by my body, I splurged often and continually abandoned my good intentions.

50% mind / 50% body:

There were some years when I had really great will-power and felt that food-centered burdens weren't a major focus in my life. When tempted by desserts, I could be strong and walk away regularly. When choosing a portion size, I could be conservative in spite of how good the food looked because I knew it meant fewer calories. I seemed to have everything under control and was relatively content. But really, I was simply holding the war at bay, because the root of the issue had not yet been addressed.

The 50/50 balance felt much better. However, when it came to choosing what to put in my mouth, the strain of the emotional tug of war still lingered.

10% mind / 90% body:

This is a comfortable place to be. For breakfast today I had oats and milk with a pinch of brown sugar. As I thought about what to eat, I subconsciously desired to feel good, full, and fueled. This is what I came up with—yum. On another day I may have chosen eggs and toast or whole grain waffles with fruit. The common thread, however, is that my choices focus on feeling fueled, not the pleasure of a sugar rush nor the counting of calories.

> My choices focus on feeling fueled, not the pleasure of a sugar rush nor the counting of calories.

I know that licorice doesn't exactly fit the "make you feel fueled" filter, but I also don't believe in absolutes. A couple of weeks ago I was craving licorice, so I bought some. Several pieces hit the spot, but while those around me continued to indulge, I stopped with very little difficulty as my body gave me about three or four bites of warning, suggesting that any more would make me feel "sort of sick like." It wasn't a hard choice because now my *body* has significantly more influence when it comes to what I eat than does my *mind*. I enjoyed the licorice until my body said "enough." Then I stopped and didn't beat myself up for tapping in to that 10% of my emotional persuasion. It was tasty.

These three simple comparisons are just that—simple. Of course there are numerous levels in between, but which person do you identify with most? Where would you like to be? Following the principles outlined in *Stop Thinking about It* is what gradually converted me from heavily favoring the will of my mind's appetite, to heavily favoring that of my body, and the difference was staggering.

Summary: When we choose what to eat, we consider what our mind wants and what our body wants, each bearing varied influence when it comes down to our choice. Listening to our body's physical cues will naturally tip the scale of influence heavily in favor of good health.

CHAPTER 4

Using Food as a "Quick Joy"

Life is hard work—emotionally, physically, financially, spiritually. Just getting through is tough. Some sorrows are a result of our choices, and some simply come along with day-to-day living. Generally speaking, we can't control what difficulties come our way, but one thing we can always control is how we react to them. While I won't attempt to suggest that I have a solution that might take away all sorrow, I would like to look, for a moment, at what seems to be a common Band-Aid for festering emotional wounds. In an effort to escape feeling sadness or disappointment, many of us choose to satisfy our *mind's* interest in "quick joy" through food.

The initial taste of ice cream or anything tantalizing gives a "quick joy." When life leaves you feeling crummy and seems beyond your control, eating ice cream and perhaps feeling a bit of "joy" is *within* your control. The brief delight of the ice cream, though only short-lived, changes your mood for a moment.

We've all felt this before. Enjoying our favorite cookie may give us a short zing of joy. Maybe a handful of chocolate briefly sends us to a happy place. Perhaps salty foods clear our mind. Each of us has our favorites. But we know that the sweet taste only lasts a moment. We know that the sugar it contains leaves us feeling sluggish. We know the undesirable consequences of eating high calorie foods. Eating when we're down is an easy habit to form. Like an addictive drug, we return to food in upsetting times.

Does this pattern sound familiar? Do you find yourself eating between meals when you aren't necessarily hungry? Do you notice that you snack simply because you are bored? Do you pay a great deal of attention to meal times and spacing, or think about what's for dinner right after lunch? How about whether your appetite flows in accordance with your moods?

Please consider that many of us eat more than we need because we have too many happiness voids. When you find yourself snacking just because it sounds good, stop and ask yourself, "What's going on?" "Is something bothering me?" "Am I trying to dull some emotional pain?" Only *you* know the answer. Do some soul searching. Is there a deeper issue that needs to be addressed? What leaves you lacking? What is causing such routine sorrow? Ask yourself some very specific questions. Be honest with yourself. Then work toward resolving the root concerns.

> Many of us eat more than we need because we have too many happiness voids.

In the meantime, identify new or existing hobbies. What makes you smile and get excited about life? My suggestion is that you stop thinking about food and find better sources of "quick joy."

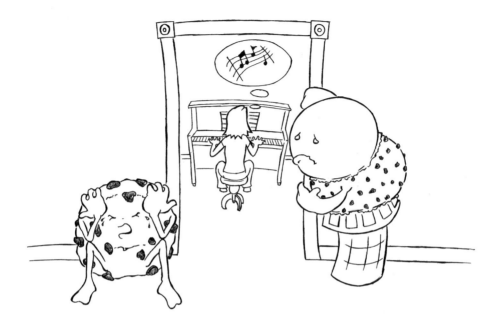

To begin, think of activities that you really like doing, things that bring immediate satisfaction. My personal favorites are to sing, play the piano, work on a project, or re-arrange the furniture in a room. Below are some examples, but I encourage you to think of what comes to mind according to *your* interests and desires.

- Recite a poem or scripture
- Read a book
- Run around the block
- Ride a bike
- Call a friend
- Water your flowers
- Take some photos
- Plan an event

- Listen to or sing a song
- Draw
- Check your email
- Put on some makeup
- Make something pretty
- Swing on a swing
- Brush your teeth
- Play the piano
- Work on a project
- Chop some wood
- Wear your favorite clothes
- Re-arrange the furniture in a room
- Clean something
- Shoot some hoops
- Check out the sports highlights

What makes you feel alive? Select one or two things to keep in your mind as your default "quick joy." So when you are burdened and feel tempted to eat for emotional reasons, these alternate activities will be recalled automatically. Initially, it may not be immediately obvious when you need to put your new "quick joy" into action. But as you become more and more aware of when you eat as a result of a negative emotion, it will be easier to recognize.

I remember a time when I was feeling burdened by the monotony of my schedule as a homemaker. I love my role as a mother and wouldn't change it for anything, but I was in a bit of a funk, feeling discouraged about my daily list of tasks. I found myself craving many more treats and snacks than were good for me. Because I was aware of my need for quality "quick joy," I was able to think beyond my situation. I needed a project. I needed something to divert my mind to a constructive activity. That week I painted a piece of old furniture. Updating furniture or building lovely things is exciting for me so it was a perfect diversion. I dove into it, really enjoyed it, and it gave me an opportunity to escape the emotional tug of war I was previously tied to. I forgot

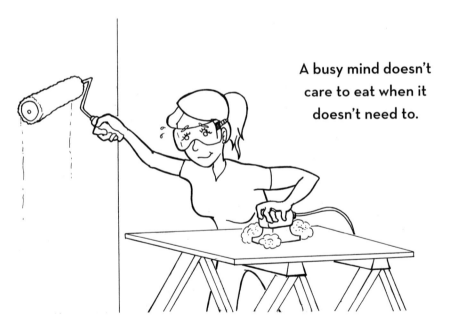

A busy mind doesn't care to eat when it doesn't need to.

about food and my concerns. As for my discouragement, it faded as I worked on creating a better balance in my routine.

When you get stuck thinking about food and find it really hard to fight it, STOP. Drop those thoughts and DO something else. A *busy* mind doesn't care to eat when it doesn't need to.

Don't get me wrong. We don't need to classify food as a symbol of weakness. Not only must we eat in order to stay alive, but as our culture suggests, food ought to be enjoyed. If you crave a banana split, go ahead and have one. Take pleasure in it. Then stop thinking about it. There's nothing wrong with enjoying the occasional forbidden favorite unless it becomes a Band-Aid for your struggles.

Summary: We all want "quick joy" from time to time. Instead of reaching for food, pick a replacement activity and do it.

CHAPTER 5

Learn About Healthy
Eating Habits

An active interest in choosing healthy foods is
a critical component to wellness. When we are
concerned about being physically healthy, giving close
attention to foods that are good for us is natural. We
tend to care about which options have fewer calories,
greater nutritional content, higher fiber, and/or offer the
best energy. In order to maintain healthy eating habits,
we must understand the benefits and drawbacks to what

we eat. This is an important part of making selections that leave us feeling fueled.

While I'm not going to pretend to be a nutritionist, and I encourage you to do your own research, I've summarized *my* basic tips for healthy eating below. Remember not to be stressed about everything you eat. Let your knowledge be a guide and not a steadfast rule.

Use whole grain flour more than white flour.

Eating whole grains and foods made with whole grain flour provides us with more nutrients and fiber than we get from refined, processed foods. Consequently, they allow us to feel better and perform at a higher capacity.

You may be familiar with the saying, "Grains are the staff of life." I hear truth in this phrase, but fluffy, white French bread and light, white biscuits aren't really that *source of life* that should be sought after. In white flour, the original wheat kernel has been stripped of the rich value it originally contained in order to create a soft, fluffy product. *Whole grains* offer strength and energy. *They* are the "staff of life." Don't misunderstand. Whole wheat sugar cookies and pie crust don't seem to be an even trade when it comes to the white flour/ wheat flour substitution, but in other baked goods, such as oatmeal chocolate chip cookies and brownies, the swap is barely detectable. Whole grain bread is delicious and satisfying. I recommend substituting wheat flour for white flour often when baking. It would be unreasonable to suggest that we never eat white flour, but try not to have it as often as whole grain products.

There are numerous grains that many people have never heard of. Quinoa, millet, amaranth, spelt, and teff are a few. Many of these grains have nutritional benefits superior to the common grains such as wheat, rice, and oats. Consider the history of amaranth, an uncommon, yet accessible grain that is high in essential amino acids, is easily digested, and is rather versatile when it comes to preparation.

Anciently, the Aztecs believed that amaranth could give a man great strength. In fact, they thought "eating a steady diet of [it] could produce a race of supermen."[3] This grain has an intriguing history.

"Not only was amaranth grown to be given to the emperor Montezuma by the tons, it was also used for religious practices. It was a source of energy and fortitude and was as important to the Aztecs as the corn and beans that kept them alive.

"Montezuma and the Aztecs' amaranth practice came to an end when Hernando Cortez observed their doings and he was so offended that he had every field of blooming amaranth burned—from the Gulf of California to the Bay of Campeche. Not only did he burn the amaranth, but those caught using it had their hand cut off. With the pillage of the

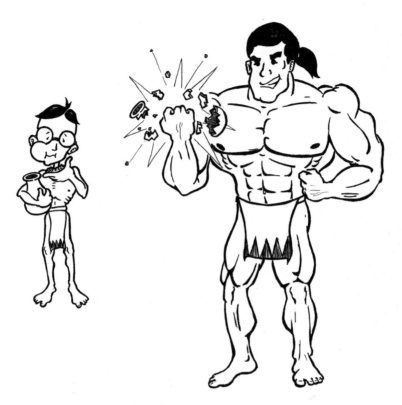

amaranth fields, historians say, came the end of the Aztec empire. Stripped and deprived of their 'power food,' warriors were left dispirited with nothing more to do but become peasants without a leader or a focus."[4]

Amaranth is only one of many less popular, yet valuable, grains. Also consider barley (high in protein, niacin, thiamine and potassium; perfect for soups and breakfast cereal), millet (a complete protein and high in iron; great substitute for white rice), quinoa (high in calcium, phosphorus, and protein; termed the "super grain" and great with cinnamon and milk), spelt (similar to wheat, but lighter, easier to digest, and more nutrient dense), and teff (a powerful, tiny grain; easy to "hide" in many dishes). These intriguing grains, and many more, can be found in whole foods stores and online vendors today with not so much as a hand to be lost upon their consumption.

Eat lots of fruits and vegetables. Fruits and vegetables are generally low in calories and nutrient dense. They cause us to feel well and contribute a great deal to a body that functions properly—period.

Eat something raw with each meal. We need enzymes for digestion, and raw foods are full of them. After they are cooked to around 118 degrees Fahrenheit, however, those enzymes are deactivated, resulting in our body's use of enzymes produced in the pancreas and other organs. Over time, given a shortage of enzymes supplied through the foods we eat, our organs become worn out, causing a significant strain on our body.

I'm not suggesting that we never eat anything cooked or processed. Just make an effort to eat something raw with each meal.

Avoid additives and preservatives. When I was in college, I remember trying to eat mostly "fat free" foods for a while. I bought fat free cream cheese, fat free deli meat, fat free yogurt, etc. I lost a few pounds over it, but it didn't last. This approach was flawed. First of all, my plan was essentially a diet, and as we've discussed previously, diets don't last. Second, when I considered the ingredient list in those unnaturally fat free foods, I found a long list of ingredients that I'd never heard of. Some of these fabricated supplements may be harmful for the body.

As a general rule, foods that are closer to their natural state will be better for you. Fast food and processed frozen dishes are generally full of additives and preservatives that slow us down. Be choosy. When grocery shopping, buy the sour cream that has three ingredients, not the one that lists nine. Pick the ice cream that has ingredients you recognize, not the one that lists a series of chemicals. Our bodies like natural foods. Of course it would be wonderful if we ate everything that was made from scratch, using only the purest of ingredients, but that's usually not practical. There are a lot of easy changes, however, that we can make with our meals simply by looking more closely at different brands and the ingredients listed on the packaging.

Fats are not entirely bad. Our body needs *some* fat. We just need to learn to recognize the right kinds of oils that offer elements of goodness and are not entirely harmful. Monosaturated, polyunsaturated, and omega-3 fats are among those that are considered "healthy." I happen to eat a lot of avocados and cook mainly with extra virgin olive oil, both of which fall into this category of "healthy" fats. The following are also sources of the same: nuts, seeds, peanut oil, canola oil, vegetable oils, cold-water fish, flax oil, and walnuts.

Snacking right before a meal will cause you to ruin your appetite. When we're hungry going into a meal, we're more likely to eat foods that will be useful for our body instead of junk food that is high in taste, but low in natural energy. Now sugar-packed foods sound awful when I'm hungry. Through listening to my body's cues, I learned that I would rather be hungry than eat a cookie on an empty stomach. My body has taught me that it doesn't want sugar or empty calories when hungry. It wants a salad with the works or meat and potatoes. It wants a huge plate of tasty veggies and chicken. Aah.

Cook with flavor. I've realized that when I reach for junk food, it's because I'm craving a bit of zip. They tend to be salty, rich, or sweet. Take a look at your recipes. Are they bland? Are they boring? Are you sick of them? Experiment with a variety of herbs and spices. You might be surprised at just how much parsley, basil, oregano, garlic, thyme, chives, rosemary, and/or sage can draw greater satisfaction from your dishes.

Today I felt "snacky." I wanted something tasty, something good. BBQ chips, candy, and soda really tempted me, but experience proved that eating them would leave me feeling uncomfortable and de-energized. I remembered that I was actually reaching for flavor. So I loaded my plate with leftover wild rice, some random shredded veggies, and homemade ranch dressing. That wasn't all, however. I have a garden that actually decided to be productive. So I snipped some Italian parsley and spinach and added it to my plate. The parsley added a tremendous burst of flavor to the whole meal, and it satisfied my craving.

Make it a point to prepare or buy meals that have great natural flavor. I'm choosing not to list recipes because the fact of the matter is there's no miracle menu. Simply weave this into your real life.

Healthy foods don't have to taste like cardboard or grass if you don't want them to. Look beyond salt, sugar, and butter. There's a whole world of sweet-and-savory, nutritious dishes that will zing your taste buds.

> There's no miracle menu. Simply weave these principles into your real life.

Drink a lot of water. "Adults are between 45 percent and 65 percent water. Only oxygen is more essential than water in sustaining the life of all organisms."[5] Over time I've naturally grown to prefer water, or water with lemon, during my meals. It doesn't interfere with the taste of what I'm eating, and I feel better after drinking it.

We should eat *many* healthy foods, not necessarily *only* health foods. Eating healthy options most of the time allows those exceptions to be a bit of a wash. Food should be enjoyed. Have a hot fudge sundae occasionally. Enjoy fried chicken once in a while. Welcome it and don't beat yourself up after you've eaten it. Simply stop thinking about it. You can enjoy your forbidden favorites in balance with the rest. The goal is not to live by absolutes, but rather to eliminate the emotional battle that so easily manipulates our choices.

Through the years I've become increasingly open-minded to new foods as I've learned about their nutritional value. Some of my slightly odd favorites are an avocado with salt, hummus served on carrot sticks, raw oats with milk (and a pinch of brown sugar), raw almonds, whole wheat bread, sweet potatoes, kale-laced fruit smoothies, whole wheat (or spelt) oatmeal chocolate chip cookies, and raw jicama prepared like a carrot stick. So try a variety. You never know what you might learn to love too.

Summary: Educate yourself about the health benefits and flaws for a variety of foods. Don't over think it, worry about it, or force it. Just become educated, knowing that if you want to be healthy, you'll need to eat plenty of healthy foods.

CHAPTER 6

We Need to Be Active

Our bodies need exercise in some form or another. Regardless of what we eat, or what we look like, our muscles need to move. There is no secret way around it. Before you write this off as what *other* people do, allow yourself to be open to options. I am not suggesting that you have to be in the gym for an hour every day or you're destined to fail. Let's be real. What works for you and your schedule? Everyone has ten minutes a day. Even a short amount of time is valuable.

There are limitless ways to be active. My many years of regular exercise have opened me to a variety of workouts. An experience that always brings a smile to my face took place while I was in high school. When I was seventeen, I worked out with aerobics tapes regularly. I'm talking about Jane Fonda, Cindy Crawford, and countless others. I had several to choose from, but after a while I got tired of them and craved a studio setting.

I decided it was worth my hard earned money to try out a nearby Jazzercise studio. In case you are unfamiliar with this type of facility, the target audience is not exactly seventeen-year-old girls. If I had to guess, it was designed to interest women who were older than me—much older. Nonetheless, they offered the right price and the right location so I didn't let a little quirkiness stand in the way of something that sounded interesting to me. Sure enough, I spent my workouts rubbing elbows with ladies that seemed to be three or four times my age.

I continued to go for several weeks. I stepped, lunged, lifted, and grapevined, while sticking out like a sore thumb. Results? Sure. Experience? Yes. Variety?

Definitely. My only regret was that I didn't splurge on the "popular" neon spandex leotard with contrasting Lycra biker shorts to match. *Maybe next time.*

Do you prefer to walk, run, bike, swim, play sports, lift weights, dance, or hike? What's interesting to you and requires you to move? If it requires movement, it can be called exercise.

Over the years, many different interests have become part of my exercise plans. I've listed a few below.

- I walked around the block for forty-five minutes pulling my children in a wagon, while talking with a friend.

- I ran wind sprints across my tiny backyard about a million times.

- I did push-ups and sit-ups every night for months at a time.

- I took tap classes.

- I stretched for one minute before going to bed.

- I ran a ten-minute loop around my neighborhood, getting back before my husband left for work in the morning.

- I did workout videos in my family room.

- "P90X: Extreme Home Fitness," I have to say, has brought the best and quickest results of anything. After having six children, I thought sit-ups were a thing of the past, but this proved me wrong in a hurry.

Again, even small amounts of exercise time, done diligently, will lend results. Obviously, with greater time and effort come greater results, but don't forget that it's important to *not* beat yourself up over your failures. Just create a doable plan, and do it the best you can.

Keep in mind that genetics determines how your healthy body will look, because some things, quite simply, are outside of your control. Instead of trying to achieve a specific set of measurements, aim for general good health and strength. After all, it feels so good to be strong.

Personally, I start squirming when anyone, in any fashion, suggests that I go work-out or encourages me to exercise. I resent it. In no way do I feel motivated unless *I* decide I am ready, *I* make the plan, and *I* want to feel better. Fitness is all about you and your personal well-being. So decide for yourself that you want to exercise for *you*, not because someone *else* wants you to. Once this occurs, you'll be one step closer to success.

> **Decide for yourself that you want to exercise for *you*, not because someone *else* wants you to.**

Don't worry about the effects of exercise before or while exercising. To be more specific, don't go into a workout thinking about how much weight you need to lose. Don't feel discouraged that it will take long to lose it. Don't think about how many calories you're burning.

Don't think that you've tried it before and it doesn't work for you. Don't sulk about how long it's going to take to finish your workout.

While you are doing sit-ups, don't think about the rolls on your stomach that are compressing in and out like an accordion. Don't even imagine what your future body will look like. When you're finished, don't weigh yourself. *Simply accomplish the task.* Make this a matter of obedience to yourself. Follow through with your plan for the day and move on.

> **Don't worry about the effects of exercise before or while exercising. Simply accomplish the task.**

Dismissing the emotional battle that plagues workouts is vital in reaching your goals. Your plan will work when you decide to get rid of that voice inside that resents your efforts, is critically aware of short term results, or says it is too hard. Drop it. Change is *change,* and you can do hard things.

Feed yourself encouraging thoughts about your plan. I've listed some examples below.

- "I really do feel good after I exercise."

- "I can do hard things."
- "This is only ten minutes and then I have the whole rest of the day to look forward to other things."
- "In twenty minutes I will have either followed through with my plan or I will not have."
- "Even if I only work out for a few minutes, I will still feel better than if I did nothing."
- "This may not be as hard as I thought."
- "I think I may actually enjoy this."
- "My plan is doable."
- "I can reach my goals."

When it comes time to carrying out your plan, at some point your old thoughts of resistance will tempt you to quit. Drop the thought. Again, as simple as it seems, change is *change*. If you want different results, you will have to *do* something different. Just pick up your feet and start.

Summary: People need exercise. Make a plan, no matter how small, and do it one day at a time.

————— ❧ —————

CHAPTER 7

Being Happy

The emotional battle surrounding food and weight loss all comes down to being happy. We worry about food, its effects, and our shape because we think that we will be truly happy if, and when, we are thin. It feels great to be healthy, and following the steps I've outlined will likely have a tremendous impact, but happiness doesn't come from being thin. We are happy as we feel inner peace and self-worth.

My burden began on that single day as a teenager when I decided that I was no longer content with how

I looked. It was then that I started supporting negative thoughts about my self image in connection with my worth. The state of our body should never control our self-worth, and unfortunately I linked the two. It wasn't until I separated them and changed the way I approached each *individually* that I was able to have peace of mind.

> **The state of your body should never control your self-worth.**

Chapters One through Six have addressed how changing the way we think can affect the state of our body. As for self-worth and lasting happiness, I believe in God and He has a significant role in my life. I know He wants us to be happy. He inspires thoughts that encourage us to feel positive self-worth and progress. Beating ourselves up over food and dieting and constantly focusing on our weight gnaws away at our positive self-worth. On the other hand, supporting positive thoughts encourages peace.

> *"As [a man] thinketh in his heart, so is he."*
> —Proverbs 23:7 [6]

The emotional battle is real. Good versus evil. Easy versus hard. Truth versus fiction. When we allow discouraging thoughts, we do so at the expense of our happiness. We all have imperfections that seem to glare at us, and our successes can take the backseat if we allow it. To which will we give greater heed? So the battle begins.

Our mind feeds our attitude and habits, but we are not subject to it; rather, our thoughts are malleable. We'll want to shape them, once we realize they truly shape us.

I remember a character on television several years ago whose name was Stewart Smiley. He was part of a comedy sketch on "Saturday Night Live."

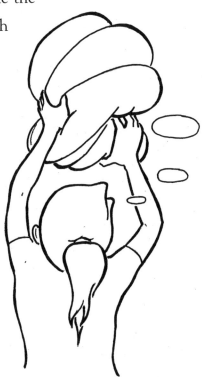

We'll want to shape our thoughts, once we realize they truly shape us.

Stewart was the king of positive self-talk—to a fault. In his skits, he listed several awful things that were going on and rejoiced in the end as he said, "But dog gone it, people like me!" I can still picture his confused look and crazy expressions. He was made to look silly and was certainly a joke, but the concept behind positive self-talk is a valid, helpful, and under-utilized principle that really does have a weighty place when it comes to the power of positive thinking.

Consider taking time to list some positive phrases in relation to your self-worth. Read them regularly. *Our attitude about everything starts with our perception of what is real.* It's always our choice as to what we base our value upon. We need not surrender our attitude to those negative thoughts that bind us to suffering.

Our attitude about everything starts with our perception of what is real.

I've listed some examples of positive phrases on the following page. Choose the ones that resonate with you, and supplement with your own as they apply.

- I can do hard things.
- Hard things bring greater satisfaction than easy things.
- I can focus my thoughts on the positive.
- I have gifts and talents specific to me.
- I am irreplaceable.
- I do many things very well.
- God knows and loves me.
- I can learn to love myself.
- I'm glad to be alive.
- I enjoy learning.
- I am ready to deal with my feelings.
- I'm happy for other people's successes.
- Blaming others doesn't bring joy.
- I can create the good in my life that I crave.
- The person I seek is seeking me too.
- I can forgive myself.
- I'm ready to experience positive change.
- Change means change, and I can do it.

Listen to positive thoughts. Drop negative ones. Do this diligently and your heart, your attitude, and your desires will change!

In my home hangs the phrase "I'm happy because . . ." Often when I'm sad, frustrated or feeling self-pity, I rehearse "I'm happy because . . ." and fill in the blank repeatedly with a different response each time.

> Drop negative thoughts. Do this diligently and your heart, your attitude, and your desires will change!

The experiences that surface are those that recently gave me even a flicker of joy, hope, or positive attention. In so doing, a little rush of happiness is brought back—one after another. This collection of fleeting positive experiences changes me. I actually *become* happier.

The bottom line is happiness. Everyone is looking for it. And being happy and being thin are two separate interests. For both individually, however, it is helpful to understand that when we control our thoughts—and we can—we may be surprised at how our outcome changes too.

Summary: The pressure we undertake to look a certain way comes down to being happy, but the state of our body should never control our self-worth. Being happy and being thin are two separate interests. For both, however, it is helpful to understand that when we control our thoughts, we control our outcome.

Conclusion

Several years ago my relationship with a certain person in my life was suffering. I felt I had been wronged. This person was hurtful to me, as well as others, and I was upset about it. I found myself rehashing these misgivings again and again in my mind, adding fuel to the fire. I analyzed it and continued to concern myself over it for several weeks. It wasn't getting any better, and my anger toward this person grew.

In time, I came to realize that I needed to stop analyzing the situation and stop justifying my position. I decided to stop thinking about it, which meant simply dropping my thoughts on the subject. When my mind would wander back to the experience, I prompted myself to replace those thoughts with others. Sometimes it would take *doing* something else altogether in order to get my mind off it completely. This took practice, but it wasn't terribly taxing. Before long, the fire inside me waned and, in no time, my heart changed. My love and concern for this person grew, and I was soon able to focus on the positive elements of our relationship again.

Whether referring to my attitude or what I do on a daily basis, the concept is the same. My thoughts have a direct relationship with my actions. It was from the above experience that the whole concept behind *Stop Thinking about It* began. My thoughts were determining my attitude. Simply dropping my negative thoughts about a person or situation naturally changed my demeanor toward them.

I had reason to believe that this example could help me gain greater peace in relation to my food-centered awareness. As mentioned in Chapter One, I tried to stop thinking about food unnecessarily, as well as any other thoughts that were contributing to my critical self-image. I never imagined that so much would snowball from this experience. What happened in response to this small step changed my life.

I once attended a party where I overheard a couple of conversations that tugged at my heart. These conversations reinforced my desire to share my experience. In one case, a woman who has battled weight issues for many years was talking among friends saying, "I just need to stay within 1,200 calories a day. I just need to do it."

At the same event, I noticed another woman who was lingering near the refreshment table. "I just love food so much," she said before putting another brownie in her mouth. The presence of tasty treats seemed to emotionally consume her, much like a common addiction.

I ached due to the emotional encumbrance these ladies placed on themselves. The burden they seemed to carry appeared significant, and I wanted them to somehow understand what I've experienced.

Having a constant, critical self-image is a tremendous burden that no one should have to endure. The messages I've shared in this book are simply based on my experience. I have been careful not to make my description any more than that. There is no magic in these pages, nor any *revolutionary breakthrough*, but it works. As I compare my emotions from before I adopted this philosophy to my mindset of recent years, the difference is unmistakable. While I still care about my figure, it doesn't worry me any longer. Clarity has replaced the cloud. My mind is free for other quality pursuits and, as it turns out, I'm the lightest I've been in years.

For me, this simply made sense. I believed it. The application was practical, and it didn't take long before their practice seemed second nature. It became part of me.

If you feel overwhelmed or disbelieving, simply take a step back and look clearly at the summaries presented in each chapter. These summaries comprise a collection of meaningful principles that complement each other well. Just try one. Take one suggestion and then come back for more.

- Stop thinking about food. Drop your thoughts about food unless you are planning dinner, buying groceries, preparing a meal, or eating. The goal is to take the emotional battle out of healthy eating.

> "After applying this approach for a week, I'm already so much happier."
> — Julie E.

- Decide that you care more about how you feel than how you look. Teach yourself to become more aware of what food choices make you feel good and which ones make you feel not so good. You'll naturally care more about fueling your body instead of telling yourself what you should or shouldn't eat, thereby either losing weight, maintaining a healthy body or both.

- When we choose what to eat, we consider what our mind wants and what our body wants, each bearing varied influence when it comes down to our choice. Listening to our body's physical cues will naturally tip the scale of influence heavily in favor of good health.

- We all want "quick joy" from time to time. Instead of reaching for food, pick a replacement activity and do it.

- Educate yourself about the health benefits and flaws for a variety of foods. Don't over think it, worry about it, or force it. Just become educated, knowing that if you want to be healthy, you'll need to eat plenty of healthy foods.

- People need exercise. Make a plan, no matter how small, and do it one day at a time

- The pressure we undertake to look a certain way comes down to being happy, but the state of our body should never control our self-worth. Being happy and being thin are two separate interests. For both, however, it is helpful to understand that when we control our thoughts, we control our outcome.

It is my hope that many of you will join me in choosing to follow this pattern for wellness and win the emotional battle surrounding food and weight loss once and for all. The last several years have been a witness to me that these principles of emotional and physical health can become a fixed way of life. *Stop Thinking about It* is a reality shift that truly *can* last a lifetime.

END NOTES

1. Sara Israelsen-Hartley, "All Women May Fear Getting Fat," Deseret News, April 15, 2010, A1 and A9.

2. Melinda Beck, "Eating to Live or Living to Eat?" Wall Street Journal, July 13, 2010, D1 and D7.

3. Brad E. Petersen, Cooking With Chef Brad, (Grass Valley: Memory Maker Productions, 2003), 11.

4. Ibid.

5. John D. Kirschmann, and Nutrition Search, Inc, Nutrition Almanac, (New York: McGraw Hill, 2007), 85.

6. Proverbs 23:7.